Low Carb Diets

The Essential Guide to Weight Loss and Health Improvement

Jennifer Schwarz

Copyright © All rights reserved worldwide.

DISCLAIMER

Note that the contents here are not presented by a medical practitioner and that any and all healthcare planning should be done under the guidance of your own medical and health practitioners. The content within only presents an overview based upon research for educational purposes and does not replace medical advice from a practicing physician.

Further, the information in this manual is provided "as is" and without warranties, either express or implied. Under no circumstances, including but not limited to negligence, shall the seller/distributor of this information be liable for any special or consequential damages that result from the use of, or the inability to use, the information presented here.

Table Of Contents

INTRODUCTION TO LOW-CARB

Many individuals use diets to deal with weight problems and improve health. According to official figures, although around 65% of Americans are overweight, just 38% are taking action.

A recent National Health Institute poll found that a third of overweight Americans attempting to lose weight are doing so by eating fewer carbohydrates (carbs), largely due to the rising popularity of fad diets like the Atkins Diet and the South Beach Diet.

Although there have undoubtedly been other low-carb or low-sugar eating regimens, and more will appear, let's look at one now.

The fundamentals of many of the big initiatives. Let's examine how they function in the modern world because learning how to do so while living in this fast-paced world would be excellent, even if it could be nice to reduce the body's sugar level and be healthier.

Dietary food budgeting, planning, preparation, and purchasing are difficulties that may become significant causes of stress and grounds for dieting failure in the age of instant messaging, rapid

Internet contact, and the already complex daily demanding schedules. With multiple jobs, dependents (both elderly and minors), and trying to fund and balance continuing education into their lives, budgets, and daily routines, dual-income families on the go and other extremely busy wage earners and dieters frequently already experience more than their fair share of daily stressors.

Simpler answers are what people need and desire. They also need simpler eating strategies. Don't waste your money on expensive, difficult-to-find gourmet goods. Forget about wasting hours on dinner preparation. Also, disregard measuring, weighing, and counting the materials.

A low-carb diet either works or doesn't work in daily life. Let's first look at some fundamental concepts and terminologies to better grasp the science underlying low-carb diets. Let's see how the plans of several of the big players fare.

Please note that the information given here is not from a medical professional and that all dietary decisions should be made with the help of your medical professionals. This information does not replace medical advice from a licensed physician; it just provides overviews of low-carb studies for educational reasons.

LOW CARB, SLOW CARB

Carbohydrates come in two basic varieties: simple and complex. Some call them rapid and slow digesting carbohydrates, harmful and good carbs, and other terminologies that may be unclear. Here is the skinny.

EASY CARBS

Most of the time, foods with simple or refined carbs have poor nutritional counts and high glycemic indexes. They digest quickly and may produce a rapid rise in blood sugar followed by a sharp decline in a short period. Health experts advise limiting these meals to keep the body functioning steadily and healthily.

White bread, potatoes, bananas, sweet delights like cookies, candies, cupcakes, cakes, and soda drinks like famous cola brands are a few examples of these simple carbohydrates.

DIFFICULT CARBS

Complex carbohydrate foods have a low to

moderate glycemic index and are packed with nutrients. These foods' higher fiber content results in delayed digestion, which is better for the body. And health professionals believe that these meals are wise choices.

Whole grains, most fruits, and vegetables are a few examples of these complex carbohydrates. Plants from the pea or bean family, known as legumes, also fall within this group.

WHICH IS BEST?

Low-carb diets may aid in weight reduction, according to studies like one published in January 2004 by the University of Arkansas for Medical Sciences; however, carbohydrates must be complex and low in glycemic index. Notably, simple carbohydrates don't have to be avoided entirely, either. In other words, as long as it's in moderation and has been allowed by your health care provider or dietary counselor, the occasional indulgence should be alright.

A side benefit of not having sugar decay from simple carbs build up on your teeth is that they will be healthier. Therefore, better bodies will reflect healthier smiles.

ADDITIONAL USEFUL TERMS

Here are more phrases to help you understand the science and health concerns about low-carb dietary planning strategies. Please note that these are merely basic concepts and that you may expand your understanding by exploring additional resources at your convenience.

Respective functions inside the body's immune system.

CALORIE

Calories are a unit of heat. A calorie may also refer to measuring the energy that comes from food for the body. In other words, the body needs more energy to absorb nutrients when the diet has more calories.

CARBOHYDRATE

A carbohydrate is one of the three main nutrients that provide the body with energy. Either single sugars or bound strings of sugar make up carbohydrates.

Sucrose, also known as table sugar, fructose, fruit sugar, and lactose, often dairy sugar, are examples of single sugars (simple carbs). Starches are often used to describe bound strings of sugar or complex carbohydrates in plants.

Wheat flour and potato starch are two examples of complex carbohydrates that are easily absorbed. Celery cellulose is one example of a non-digestible substance. The body turns carbohydrates into sugar, which is then utilized as fuel. Unused carbohydrates are turned into fat by the body.

FAT

One of the three main food types that provide the body with energy is fat. Animal or plant sources of oil are the sources of fat. The body converts it into more easily metabolized fats, either burnt off or stored.

FRUCTOSE

Sugar produced from plants, particularly maize, called fructose, is used to sweeten prepared dishes and commercial food items like sodas. The term "high-fructose corn syrup" is often used to describe this component, which first became widely popular in the 1970s.

GLUCOSE

Blood sugar is a term used to describe glucose. The body breaks down all carbs, simple or complex, into sugar, the type of sugar in the blood. The primary trigger for insulin release is the amount of glucose in the blood.

GLUCAGON

The pancreas secretes the hormone glucagon, which induces fat cells to release their glucose reserves for use as fuel. For the body to release and break down body fat, glucagon must be released. If blood sugar and insulin levels are high, the pancreas will not release glucagon because it cannot release both hormones effectively.

GLYCOGEN

Animals generally store carbohydrates as glycogen found in the liver and muscle tissue. When the body needs glucose to meet its energy demands, it does so easily. Likewise known as animal starch.

GLUCOSE INDEX

The glycemic index calculates how fast certain meals may cause your blood sugar levels to rise.

INSULIN

The body's primary metabolic hormone, insulin, is one of the two hormones the pancreas produces. The pancreas releases insulin as blood glucose levels rise to assist in transferring glucose into cells for cellular energy.

Additionally, insulin promotes the conversion of excess amino acids into protein, which is then stored in the muscle, as well as the storage of excess glucose in fatty tissue. It facilitates the storage of excess glucose as glycogen in the liver. Insulin may increase cholesterol levels, lead to fluid and salt retention, and prevent the breakdown of fat accumulated in the body. Having insufficient insulin or not enough

Diabetes may result from sensitivity to insulin's actions in the body.

RESISTANCE TO INSULIN

Insulin resistance develops when the body does not adequately react to and digest the insulin it produces. The pancreas produces too much insulin as a result of insulin resistance. The Drs. According to Michael and Mary Eades of Protein Power, Type II diabetes, obesity, high blood pressure, raised cholesterol, and other illnesses and ailments are all brought on by insulin resistance.

KETONES

Ketones are a molecule that occurs when the body breaks down fat for energy due to insufficient glucose to meet demands and the liver's depletion of glycogen. Ketones in excess result in foul breath and are detectable in urine during strip testing.

KETOSIS

When glucose is scarce, the body enters a state of ketosis and uses stored fat as fuel. A means of surviving in times of hunger.

It is often believed to be a bad long-term condition for the body. When someone who is starving or not eating for any other reason goes into ketosis, it may lead to significant sickness and, ultimately, death.

PROTEIN

Protein is one of the three main nutritional types that provide the body with energy. Animal and soy products and certain plant products like legumes (beans, peanuts, and peas) are protein sources. Metabolized by the body into amino acids during digestion and stored as protein in muscle cells.

SUCROSE

Table sugar is another term for sucrose from sugar cane plants.

STARCH

In meals like potatoes, white rice, bread, bagels, and other items, starch, a form of sugar, may be found.

FAT TRANS

Trans fat, also known as hydrogenated or partly hydrogenated fat/oil, is a form of processed fat that does not exist naturally. Used in various processed foods, including margarine and salad dressings, and baked items, including doughnuts, breads, crackers, potato chips, and cookies.

CHAPTER 1

LOW-CARB HISTORY AND BACKGROUND

It wasn't until the USDA declared that six to eleven portions of grains and starches per day were included in the model food pyramid for America that the phrase "low-carb" was born. However, the first low-carb diet as similar to a commercial one as you could find was a tract titled Letter on Corpulence authored by William Banting in 1864, more than a century before the fashionable Atkins diet.

Banting had some crippling health issues, mostly brought on by his obesity or "corpulent" state. He looked in vain for remedies for his weight issue, which many medical professionals at the time said was an inevitable side effect of aging. He also tried eating less but kept gaining weight and had some health issues. He could not comprehend how his small quantities of food contributed to his weight issue.

Few men have been as physically and mentally active as I was during my fifty-year business career, from which I had retired. As a result, my corpulence and subsequent obesity were not caused by a lack of necessary physical activity, excessive eating or drinking, or any other form of self-indulgence, except that I indulged in the basic foods of bread, milk, butter, beer, sugar, and potatoes more freely than my peers.

Many harried modern Americans will be familiar with Banting's former unhealthy daily diet:

"My former diet consisted of bread and milk for breakfast or a pint of tea with lots of milk, sugar, and buttered toast; meat, beer, a lot of bread (which I was always fond of), and pastry for dinner; a tea meal similar to that of breakfast; and typically a fruit tart or bread and milk for supper. I slept poorly and with little comfort."

You can see how Banting's diet was so similar to the typical fast-paced modern American diet by substituting a Pop-tart, doughnut, or muffin with coffee and plenty of cream and sugar for breakfast, a fast food burger and fries with a super-sized soft drink for lunch, and a frozen pot pie or pizza for dinner followed by dessert.

When his doctor put these things on a "forbidden foods list," Banting shed 50 pounds and 13 inches in a year. He managed to keep it off and lived a long, much healthier life.

His new diet included a variety of meat dishes, as he detailed below:

For breakfast, I have five to six ounces of either beef mutton, kidneys, broiled fish, bacon, or any other cold meat, except hog or veal, along with a big cup of unsweetened tea or coffee, a small biscuit, or one ounce of dry toast, for a total of six ounces of solid food and nine ounces of fluids.

Five or six ounces of fish, except salmon, herrings, and swordfish, for supper at 2 p.m.

Or eels, any meat other than pork or veal, any vegetable other than potato, parsnip, beetroot, turnip, or carrot, one ounce of dry toast, fruit from an unsweetened pudding, any type of poultry or game, and two or three glasses of good claret, sherry, or Madeira—Champagne, port, and beer are prohibited. This amounts to ten to twelve ounces of solid food and ten ounces of liquid.

At six o'clock in the evening, I have a cup of tea without milk or sugar, two to three ounces of cooked fruit, a few rusks, and about nine ounces of drink.

At nine o'clock for dinner. A meal-sized serving of three or four ounces of meat or fish, water, and one or two glasses of claret or sherry equals four ounces of solid food and seven ounces of liquid.

If needed, a glass or two of claret or sherry or a tumbler of grog (gin, whiskey, or brandy without sugar).

His friends and acquaintances started to notice the drastic improvements in his look and health, and just like today, they were curious about his diet. Most importantly, Banting could perceive and feel the change for himself.

It may be a matter of opinion or a friendly observation. Still, I can honestly say that I feel restored in health, "bodily and mentally," I appear to have more muscular power and vigor, have a better appetite, eat and drink with a good appetite, and sleep well. I am told by everyone who knows me that my appearance improved and that I seem to bear the stamp of good health. All signs of heartburn, indigestion, and acid reflux—all of which I used to suffer from—have disappeared. Since I can now stoop with ease and freedom, I have stopped using boot hooks and other such aids, which were formerly required but are now unneeded. I no longer have the sporadic sense of dizziness, and what I consider to be a tremendous gift and comfort is that I can now safely stop wearing the knee braces that I had to wear for many years and the umbilical truss.

His how-to book on dieting was widely read and translated into other languages. But eventually, it was forgotten.

In Letter on Corpulence, Banting stated that a prevalent health dilemma of our day did not exist in his time. This was the paradox of obesity among the poor, often considered an issue of excess. The refined sugary meals that lead to weight gain could not be purchased by the impoverished in the 19th century. But in the modern day, impoverished individuals can certainly do so.

Many low-income families stretch their food budgets by buying unhealthy processed and refined meals, the writer stated in a recent Associated Press piece headlined "Health Paradox: Obesity Attacks Poor." Barbassa remarked, "Of one family,

"Due to a lack of employment throughout the winter, Caballero feeds her three children and husband the cheapest food, including potatoes, bread, and tortillas.

Foods heavy in sugar and fat have become less expensive than fruits and vegetables, and the poor are paying a steep price with rising obesity and diabetes rates.

Unfortunately, the Caballero family's poor health is caused by these inexpensive necessities. Although fresh meat, fruits, and vegetables with low levels of starch may be more costly and have a shorter shelf life, they are unquestionably worth the cost in terms of reduced medical costs and improved health.

As "calories" gained popularity over time, several methods of quantifying them were included in nutritional advice. Additionally, many other topics were investigated, such as how often and in what quantities to consume certain meals.

Although Banting's diet subsequently lost popularity, low-carb diets started to resurface in the 20th century. The Atkins and Scarsdale diets, which gained popularity in the 1970s, are the two most well-known. The Atkins diet allowed for unrestricted calorie consumption as long as those calories came from protein, fat, and vegetables, and carbohydrate intake was kept to a minimum. In contrast, Scarsdale has a defined 14-day meal plan that must be adhered to and severely limits calories.

In the 1980s, Atkins and Scarsdale lost popularity as the U. With the USDA food pyramid, the U.S. Department of Agriculture promoted the consumption of grains and grain products.

Only in the 1990s did we start to see a comeback of low-carb diets that seemed more than a trend. It's a way of life! The number of diets and shops specializing in low-carb items is growing as more and more people become aware of the potential weight reduction and other health advantages of eating low-carb.

The fundamental tenet of most low-carb diets is that eating too many simple, refined carbs causes the body to produce too much insulin, which in turn causes the body to store too much fat. The midsection is a particularly noticeable location for this fat accumulation.

While there are differences in degree across the various diets, they all concur that our bodies are negatively impacted by excessive insulin production.

CHAPTER 2

THE ROLE OF INSULIN

The body employs three fundamental energy units:

- Fats
- Proteins
- Carbohydrates

Blood glucose may be produced from all three. While carbs are metabolized fast compared to fats and proteins, this causes quick rises in the body's blood sugar levels. The pancreas produces and releases insulin in response to these blood sugar rises until the level stabilizes.

As soon as the body notices that blood sugar levels have climbed over the ideal range, insulin, a hormone produced in the pancreas that reduces blood glucose levels, is released into the blood.

The very effective hormone insulin controls the body's fuel storage mechanisms. Insulin will tell the body to store more sugar or fat in the fat cells if there is too much of either substance in the blood. Additionally, insulin instructs these cells to hold onto their fat reserves, preventing the body from using that fat as energy.

Insulin effectively halts weight loss since the body cannot release the stored fat for use as energy. The more successfully the body's insulin levels inhibit fat cells from releasing their deposits, the more challenging it is to lose weight. Numerous experts assert that elevated insulin levels have the potential to, over time, result in insulin resistance and major health issues like those mentioned below:

1. Insulin resistance and elevated insulin levels
2. Decrease in metabolism resulting in weight gain
3. A rise in adipose tissue and a decline in muscle
4. Increased aging
5. A rise in dietary intolerances and allergies
6. Stressed-out immune system
7. Increased risk of cancer, diabetes, obesity, and heart disease

The body swiftly converts carbohydrates, particularly simple ones like sugar and starch, into sucrose, which enters the bloodstream more quickly and triggers the release of a lot of insulin. The body produces less insulin and stores fewer calories as fat when consuming fewer carbohydrates. Less fat storage results in less weight gain, while eating less carbohydrates reduces insulin levels and the body's use of fat reserves as fuel.

Every low-carb diet is based on the idea that a body that generates less insulin burns fat more efficiently than one that produces much of it. A time of very low carbohydrate consumption is encouraged by certain regimens to induce ketosis and hasten the body's fat-burning process.

Typically, they are referred to as induction times. Extreme carb restriction might last anywhere from seven days to as long as it takes you to attain your goal weight. Following this time of very low carbohydrate diets, maintenance of carbohydrate intake is continued to avoid weight gain. You can consume just so much carbohydrate depending on your particular biological system. You'll likely need to do some testing to determine your optimal carbohydrate consumption.

No matter how many carbohydrates you consume, it will be less than average, and you will still avoid white flour, white floral products, and certain other starchy and sweet meals. These eating regimens are referred to as low-carb lifestyles for this reason.

In the long run, you must be prepared to give up simple carbohydrates to succeed with low-carb.

Here are the top 14 low-carb diet books and regimens, along with a brief description of what each one entails.

1. ATKINS DIET

The Atkins diet is perhaps the most well-known low-carb eating plan. The Atkins diet, developed by Dr. Robert Atkins in the 1970s, is regarded by some as the most severe low-carb eating regimen.

Dr. Atkins thought that rather than excessive eating, the majority of obesity is brought on by an overactive insulin production system. He believed that most overweight persons ate less than their slender counterparts and that carbohydrate addiction might cause overeating. But they consume the carbohydrates they want, which increases their insulin levels and slows down fat burning.

Dr. Atkins supports the ketogenic fat-burning method, which involves consuming less than 40 grams of carbs daily. To verify that they are consistently in a state of ketosis, he counsels his followers to get testing strips so they may check the level of ketones in their urine every day. He also suggests taking dietary supplements to maintain a balance between the body's systems and nutrition.

The Atkins Diet has four phases: Induction, Ongoing Weight Loss, Pre-Maintenance, and Lifetime Maintenance.

The Induction diet is relatively restrictive regarding carbohydrate intake (20 grams or fewer daily), but it is lenient regarding fat and protein intake. Low-starch veggies should be recognized as the preferred source of carbohydrates. The Ongoing Weight Loss Diet (OWL) comes after this 14-day diet phase.

Certain healthy carbohydrates may be reintroduced during the OWL phase. However, the daily intake must not exceed 40 grams. Until they attain their goal weight, dieters adhere to OWL. After achieving their goal weight, dieters move on to the Pre-Maintenance diet, where they experiment with reintroducing certain healthy carbohydrates until they identify their carb tolerance level (the total number of grams of carbs they can eat each day without gaining weight).

Dieters begin lifetime maintenance when they know how much carbohydrates they can take while maintaining their goal weight. They will avoid sweets, processed foods, white flour, and hydrogenated fats and oils at this location.

The Atkins diet permits numerous foods, and Atkins shops nationwide sell items that align with the plan.

2. DIET FOR CARBOHYDRATE ADDICTS

Drs., a husband and wife scientific duo. The phrase "carbohydrate addict" was first used by Rachael and Richard Heller in their 1993 book The Carbohydrate Addict's Diet.

According to the theory, some individuals depend on carbs, like alcoholics become dependent on alcohol, and drug addicts become dependent on narcotics. Strong cravings, insulin resistance, and weight gain are all effects of this addiction.

By the time the first book was published, Dr. Rachael Heller had sustained her substantial weight reduction for over twenty years and created the diet to cure her obesity. According to the Hellers, a carbohydrate-induced insulin imbalance makes the body seek more food and prevents serotonin from being released, which would otherwise indicate that the body is full. Overeating and weight gain result from this.

The Hellers advise carb addicts to restrict their carb consumption to one "reward meal," eat three meals a day, and refrain from snacking until they have completed the diet's weight reduction phase.

The Hellers discuss psychological factors that might lead carb addicts to binge on carbohydrates and put on weight in addition to the diet plan. They advise dieters to recognize their emotional triggers and learn how to avoid them to lose weight.

One of the key tenets of this diet is that being overweight is not the fat person's fault. Why? The person's DNA and the carbs' ability to get people addicted to them are working against them.

The Hellers advise against processed meals and various sugars, much like any other low-carb diet. However, they add that, if desired, some starchy carbohydrates should be consumed with incentive meals to increase the dieter's likelihood of long-term adherence to the diet.

According to the Hellers, carb addiction may be managed over the long term with excellent nutrition and a balanced diet, but it cannot be cured. Therefore, those addicted to carbohydrates must exercise caution to avoid future weight gain and carb binges.

3. THE HAMPTON DIET

Dr. Fred Pescatore, a former associate medical director of the Atkins Institute, created Hampton's Diet. This diet combines the best elements of the Mediterranean diet with low-carb dieting principles. He advocates consuming enough monounsaturated fats to promote weight reduction and stave against conditions including diabetes, heart disease, and cancer. The Hampton's Diet, released in May 2004 and detailed all of this, lays it out.

In his book, he urges readers to consume a lot of Australian macadamia nut oil and includes a thirty-day meal plan, gourmet recipes, and information about the oil. If you cannot afford the macadamia nut oil, which he believes to be the finest for your health, he advises using a specific cold-pressed virgin olive oil.

There are several recipes, but most are fairly gourmet in style and involve pricey components. Many of the book's recipes were developed by renowned chefs and restaurant owners whose low-carb dishes are popular with clients all over the globe.

The Atkins diet greatly influences Dr. Pescatore's diet due to his relationship with Dr. Atkins. The focus on fruits and vegetables, the use of healthy fats such as macadamia nut oil, and the recommendation that all skin and fat be removed from animals before cooking seem to be the key points of distinction.

While sharing many of Atkins' characteristics, this plan also offers excellent dishes, 30-day meal plans, and more than 100 recipes.

4. THE GLYCEMIC INDEX DIET

According to The Glycemic Index (GI) Diet, by Rick Gallop, a former president of The Heart and Stroke Foundation of Ontario, "if you can understand a traffic light, you'll understand this diet."

According to its glycemic index, food is divided into three classes by Gallop, which measures how quickly they raise blood sugar levels. He divides the food into categories marked with green, yellow, and red lights. The GI of glucose is fixed at 100, and all other foods are measured against it. Red-light foods must be avoided, yellow-light foods should only be consumed periodically during the continuing maintenance phase, and green-light foods should always be the foundation of your diet.

There is no need to buy any specialized meals. Simply check where your favorite meals fall on the menu, stick to the green, yellow, and orange food groups, and skip the red. Period. Gallop advises dieters not to begin with a crash diet and to anticipate losing one to two pounds each week. This diet encourages dieters to trim lipids in addition to carbohydrates, even though it is low in carbohydrates and has a lower protein intake than most other diets. Additionally, he promotes eating three meals a day that are balanced, including carbohydrates, proteins, and fats, and exercising for 30 minutes each day.

Gallop contends that GI diet adherents should see the diet as a lifestyle choice they will maintain for the rest of their lives. But it's not simple. For instance, take a look at this list of "Red Light foods" and observe all of the "good eats":

- Refried beans
- Baked beans with pork
- Alcoholic beverages
- Regular soft drinks and bagels.
- Cornbread
- Croissants
- Baguettes
- Cakes
- Cookies
- Kaiser rolls

- English muffins
- Hamburger buns
- Hot dog buns
- English muffins
- Doughnuts
- Pancakes
- Waffles
- Pizza
- Stuffing with regular granola bars
- White bread
- Millet
- Tortillas
- Cold Cereals
- White Rice
- Instant Rice
- Rice Cakes
- Granola with Cream of Wheat
- Grits
- Oatmeal
- Caffeine-free
- Instant oatmeal
- Croutons
- Mayonnaise
- Cheese
- Chocolate milk
- Cottage cheese Cream
- Ice cream with cream cheese
- Whole 2% milk
- Sour cream

- Yogurt
- Lard
- Peanut butter
- Hard Margarine
- Coconut oil
- Almond butter
- Tropic oils
- Regular salad dressing
- Cantaloupe
- Vegetable shortening
- Dates
- Prunes
- Honeydew melon
- Watermelon
- Raisins
- All fruit drinks
- Applesauce with sugar
- Fruit beverages in cans
- Bologna
- Bratwurst
- Sorbet
- Regular eggs
- Ground beef with 20% fat
- Hamburgers
- Pastrami
- Processed beef
- Hot dogs
- Regular bacon
- Sushi rolls

- Salami
- Pasta in cans
- Couscous
- Gnocchi
- Noodles
- Macaroni and cheese
- Alfredo sauces
- Meat or cheese-filled pasta
- Jell-O
- French fries
- Candy
- Potato Chips

5. NEANDERTHIN

NeanderThin author Ray Audette promotes his diet as a method to "Eat like a caveman to achieve a lean, strong, healthy body." Audette had rheumatoid arthritis and diabetes at the young age of 33. Audette decided to do a nutritional study to discover a better treatment after learning from physicians that his disease was manageable but not curable.

After the study, he followed a "Paleolithic" hunter-gatherer diet, similar to what our ancestors consumed before migrating to agricultural communities. His blood sugar levels returned to normal after a week; after a month, he had dropped 25 pounds, his arthritis pain had subsided, and his muscle tone had improved.

Audette asserts that compared to our agricultural Neolithic forebears, our Paleolithic ancestors were far healthier and lived longer happier lives. He claims that compared to the Paleolithic man, the Neolithic man was shorter, had worse oral health, and was more prone to obesity. In addition, women started menstruating earlier and had more children more often, which led to population growth that further supported agricultural lifestyles.

He believes that contemporary man should transition into a modern hunter-gatherer society by removing items that need human intervention to become edible. Milk, cereals, beans, potatoes, alcohol, and sugar are some of these foods. Wheat, maize, rice, oats, barley, and rye are all considered to be grains. He also believes that eating these carbohydrates would result in cravings and, ultimately, binge eating.

According to Audette's general guideline, if a fruit or vegetable may be eaten unprocessed and raw, including it in a NeanderThin diet is okay. He says many vegetables, including potatoes, are deadly if not properly kept and treated with fungicides. To assist the body in burning stored fat, he also promotes consuming fruits throughout their season and reducing consumption during the winter.

Ten commandments are given. In a nutshell, they are: Don't consume grains, beans, potatoes, dairy, sweets, fruits, veggies, nuts, or seeds. Do eat meat and fish.

6. PROTEIN STRENGTH

Drs. Audette, Michael, and Mary Eades, co-authors of The Protein Power LifePlan, think that today's health issues are brought on by our contemporary diet, which is high in grains and processed food. (It should be noted that Dr. Michael Eades wrote the preface to Audette's NeanderThin.)

The Eades' food pyramid is the USDA pyramid reversed upside down, with whole grains at the top, vegetables and fruit in the middle, and proteins at the base.

The Eades also recommend regular exercise and modified frequent sunbathing sans sunblock to assist the body in manufacturing necessary vitamins and regulating bodily systems, in addition to basing your diet on a high protein and low grain intake. They also advise daily use of a full multivitamin and mineral supplement.

Dieters must determine their minimal protein needs by height, Weight, and sex for each meal. At least that much protein should be included in every meal, and protein should be ingested during every meal. Bad fats, including maize oil, vegetable cooking oils, margarine, vegetable shortening, and any partly hydrogenated oils, should be avoided by dieters.

Phased diet implementation enables a seamless transition to a low-carb diet and reduces Weight. Carbohydrate consumption is restricted to 7 to 10 grams of each meal during the Intervention period. The Transition level, the second phase, must be followed for many months. Up to 15 net carb grams per meal are permitted at this level. Each meal may take up to 30 grams of carbohydrates during the final maintenance phase. Additionally, they provide menu options and meal plans for Purists, Hedonists, and Dilettantes, three categories of low-carb dieters.

Relying largely on animal protein and avoiding all dairy products, alcohol, caffeine, legumes, sweets (apart from honey), processed foods, cereal grains, and goods that include them, purists aim to recreate a Paleolithic eating pattern in the contemporary world. They will also consume fresh, organic fruits, vegetables, and game or natural meat products.

The biggest dietary latitude is given to hedonists. All

they need to do is consume enough protein, restrict their carbohydrate intake to a certain amount every meal, drink enough water, eat plenty of healthy fats, and take magnesium and potassium supplements.

Between these two extremes, The Dilettantes choose the moderate path. They continue to steer clear of anything made from their flours, including wheat, maize, millet, and rye. However, they are permitted organic dairy products, a small amount of natural sugar, and carbohydrates within the daily limits.

7. SCHWARZBEIN THEORY

The celebrities' go-to endocrinologist is Dr. Diana Schwarzbein. Schwarzbein, who has treated Suzanne Somers, Larry Hagman, and many others, advocates thorough hormonal testing before recommending different food and exercise regimens and targeted hormone replacement therapy to address deficits.

The Schwarzbein Principle, Dr. Schwarzbein's five-step program for achieving maximum health, outlines her eating philosophy.

Healthy Nutrition is the first phase of the program, and there are ten fundamental guidelines:

1. Never again miss a meal
2. Consume whole, unprocessed foods.
3. Consume healthy meals.
4. As the meal's primary Nutrition, choose a protein.
5. Add some beneficial fats.
6. Include actual carbs
7. Include some non-starchy veggies
8. ingest snacks
9. Consume solid food
10. Obtain enough liquids

Stress Management is the program's second stage.

1. Make it a habit to relax every day.
2. Get a perspective on your life.
3. Monitor signs of stress.
4. Obtain adequate rest.

Third, stay away from any hazardous substances, such as:

1. Nicotine
2. Alcohol
3. distilled sugar
4. Synthetic sweeteners
5. Illicit drugs
6. Additives, preservatives, and MSG
7. Fat blockers and fake fats
8. Caffeine

9. Certain prescription medicines

Fourth, engage in resistance, flexibility, and relaxation activities.

Finally, hormone replacement treatment is the last step to achieving optimum health when required.

8. SOMERSIZING

"Somersizing" was initially discussed by Suzanne Somers in 1992's Suzanne Somers Eat Great, Lose Weight. By eating a lot of healthy fats, proteins, and good carbohydrates like fruits and vegetables, you may substitute sugar and "funky foods" for them. This eating style is known as isomerizing. For food to be readily digested by the body, particular food combinations must be used. Dieters work out in two stages, with the first (Level One) intended to help them lose weight and trigger "the melt" of fat and the second (Level Two) intended to help them maintain their optimum weight over time.

Proteins/Fat, Veggies, Carbohydrates, and Fruit are the four Somersizing dietary classes that Somers divides food into. She advises eating fruit on an empty stomach. Meat, poultry, eggs, natural oils, butter, cream, and cheese are examples of proteins and fats.

Fresh veggies with little carbohydrates are vegetables. Whole-grain bread, pasta, cereals, and non-fat dairy products are carbohydrates.

The "Seven Easy Steps to Somersizing" are as follows:

1. Get rid of any foul food.
2. 20 minutes before a carbohydrate meal, one hour before a protein or fat meal, and at least two hours before the last meal consume fruit on an empty stomach.
3. Eat healthy fats and vegetables.
4. Eat carbohydrates together with vegetables.
5. Separate your pros/fats and carbs.
6. If transitioning from Pro/Fats to Carbos or vice versa, wait 3 hours between meals.
7. Do not skip meals; have at least three meals every day.

Example Of Funky Foods Include:

White Sugar
Brown Sugar
Beets
Carrots
Raw sugar
Corn syrup
Sucrose

Honey
Maple syrup
Bananas
Butternut Squash
Corn
Acorn Squash
Pumpkin
Parsnips
Potatoes
Rice
Sweet Potatoes
White Flour
Yams
Avocados
Hubbard squash
Coconuts
Liver
Whole milk
Nuts
Beer
Olives
Soy
Tea
Soda
Cocoa
Coffee
Hard Alcoholic
Wine

Every item on the Funky Foods list must be avoided during the first phase of the diet (Level One); however, during the maintenance phase (Level Two), some foods may be reintroduced in moderation. Somers market her line of synthetic.

"SomerSweet" is a brand of sweetener. She includes recipes for meals, snacks, and desserts in all her publications.

9. THE SOUTH BEACH DIET

The South Beach Diet, created by Dr. Arthur Agatston, prides itself on instructing dieters to choose the proper carbohydrates and fats. Three stages make up the diet. In the first diet, dieters suppress their appetite for harmful carbohydrates and quicken weight reduction. In the second phase, weight reduction is slower and certain forms of carbohydrates are reintroduced. The "Diet for Life" phase is the last. The dieter will continue to eat this way for the rest of their lives. The dieter simply repeats the induction and pre-maintenance periods if, at any point, he starts to gain Weight.

The first stage focuses on high-quality meat sources for protein, along with many fresh vegetables and salads dressed with genuine olive oil. During the

14-day induction period, all fruit, bread, rice, pasta, potatoes, baked goods, soy milk and cheese, yogurt, beets, carrots, and maize are prohibited. All candies, cakes, ice cream, sugar, and meats cured in molasses or sugar fall under this category.

In addition to three meals a day, the plan recommends a mid-morning and mid-afternoon snack.

There is a daily food plan as well. In the induction phase, this diet involves severe portion restrictions. 20 peanuts would be an example of a daily snack. Another snack choice is 30 pistachios.

Unlike Atkins, excessive protein intake is neither suggested nor permitted on this diet. However, some stringent portion control does loosen up as the diet progresses, and dieters can eat until they feel full.
In the second phase of the diet, some restricted items may be gradually reintroduced, perhaps in a modified form. The second phase continues until the dieter reaches their desired Weight. Products with white flour, potatoes, maize, carrots, beets, and sweet fruits like pineapple and banana are still prohibited.

Dieters go on to their Diet for Life or maintenance diet after they have reached their target weight.
Processed foods, items made with white flour, sweet fruits, and generally anything with a high glycemic

index are prohibited during this period.

Dr. Agatston anticipates a weight reduction of eight to thirteen pounds over the 14-day induction phase, with abdominal fat being the first to go. As long as they do not go crazy with the carb reintroduction, dieters should continue to lose 1-2 pounds per week in the second phase.

10. SUGAR BUSTERS!

Over at Sugar Busters! Dieters reduce sugar to lose Weight. A group of physicians and the CEO of a Fortune 500 company from New Orleans developed this diet after realizing that low-fat meals are high in sugar and that this sugar triggers an unhealthy insulin response and results in weight gain.

They emphasize enjoying delicious cuisine while avoiding some off-limits items like processed sugar and goods made from refined grains. Although it is not banned, dieters should gradually lower their sugar intake and learn to spot foods that contain hidden sugars. It is also encouraged to combine foods properly to prevent weight gain.

On this diet, you give up potatoes, maize, white rice, bread made from refined flour, most cold cereals, beets, carrots, refined sugar, corn syrup, molasses, honey, sugary colas, and beer.

The writers advise consuming fruit in its entire form and on its own whenever feasible. However, a focus is put on being able to regulate food amounts equivalent to what can comfortably fit on a typical-sized dinner plate. They allow three meals, two snacks, and a sugar-free dessert.

A 14-day diet and food plan are included at the start of the regimen. Dieters are advised to consume carbohydrates with a lower glycemic index and fiber content. The authors recommend lean, well-trimmed meats as a source of protein. They predict you will eat around 30% protein, 40% carbohydrates, and 30% monounsaturated and other fats.

11. THE ZONE

The Zone, developed by Dr. Barry Sears, promotes a balanced diet of carbohydrates and proteins. Dr. Sears advises that one portion of your plate should be reserved for protein, and the other two should be reserved for fruits and vegetables. This amounts to 30% protein, 40% carbohydrates, and 30% fat. The protein quantity for each meal should be around the size of your hand, clenched securely. Two loosely clasped fists should be the size of the carbohydrate part, and your thumb should be the size of the additional fat portion.

Measuring and controlling meal portions is central to The Zone. The "block" is another tool that Zone dieters may use to measure their intake. A dieter's daily food intake depends on the appropriate meal portion size, which should be at least 11 blocks for adults.

The protein quantities on this diet are restricted, and you can't eat until you're full. Your meal is over after consuming all of your Zone meal portions.

The fundamental Zone guidelines are to:

1. Each day, have a Zone meal within an hour after awakening.
2. Every time you eat, have a balanced meal from the Zone (protein, carbs, and fat).
3. Consume five meals and two snacks each day.
4. Never skip a Zone meal for more than five hours.
5. Increase your intake of fruits, vegetables, bread, pasta, grains, and carbohydrates.
6. Every day, consume 64 ounces of water.
7. Make your subsequent meal Zone-friendly if you make a mistake at one meal.

The Zone diet does not restrict any foods, although certain unfavorable carbohydrates should be avoided or, if consumed, should not make up more than 25% of any meal or snack. The typical suspects in the category of unfavorable carbohydrates are white flour, potatoes, sugar, white rice, juices, sodas, alcohol, bananas, grapes, carrots, maize, and coffee-containing beverages. According to Dr. Sears, eating these foods may induce hormonal imbalances, inflammation of the body's tissues, and an overall decline in health, in addition to increasing insulin production.

Packaged foods, including nutritional bars, beverages, baked goods, and supplements, are associated with the Zone diet. However, the Zone nutritional bar does include high fructose corn syrup. However, it is a "high-quality" version with a slower glycemic index than the typical type, and the protein in the bar helps to further decrease the insulin response, as stated on the company website. Consume with the utmost care.

12. THE GOOD THIN

Dr. Fred Pescatore authored the book Thin For Good: The One Low-Carb Diet That Will Finally Work for You before he started praising Australian macadamia nut oil. This program contains strategies for men and women and a low-carb diet for vegetarians and investigates the mind-body relationship in long-lasting weight reduction.

Dr. Pescatore outlines "The Eleven Emotional Levels of Eating" in her book Thin for Good. They are as follows:

1. Anger is a common emotion at the start of a new diet, which is beneficial since it serves as motivation.
2. When we compare our seeming lack of success to that of others, we might get frustrated. However, this is a negative feeling that often leads individuals to quit.
3. Sadness is frequently associated with self-pity, grief for bygone eras, and eating.
4. Fear: This feeling, which might appear simultaneously as the initial triumphs in weight reduction (can I maintain this diet for the rest of my life?), is often extremely difficult to let go of.
5. When you start to recognize and accept your unhealthy eating patterns, you must first go through the first four emotions to reach this more positive stage.
6. Trepidation is the uncertainty that might arise when you start to see the effects of your diet. It is often characterized as uneasiness, edginess, and wariness.
7. When you compare yourself to others, you might experience the negative sensation of

envy.

8. Add some diversity to your meals in line with your diet plan to avoid boredom, which may destroy a diet.
9. Joy occurs after you have accomplished actual accomplishments; try not to undermine it.
10. Relief is the start of the pleasant feelings that should be cherished.
11. Satisfaction: the last feeling felt when someone achieves their weight reduction objectives

Dr. Pescatore advises low-carb comfort food recipes and other activities to help you work through your emotions, saying that they might make you feel better while coping with these emotions.

He advises adopting the "Mind Over Calories" idea since it will let you lose weight permanently. He says that after he started losing Weight, this idea helped him keep it off. Mind Over Calories aims to teach you how to control your cravings for high-sugar, high-carb meals.

Your diet will bring you back to your previous state of being overweight and unwell.

Additionally, he offers advice on nutritional supplements for both sexes, lists of items to stay away from if you're on a yeast-restricted diet, have thyroid or hormonal issues, and offers more than 40 pages of recipes.

The Thin For Good Food Pyramid places proteins and lipids at the base, complex carbohydrates immediately above them, simple carbohydrates like starchy vegetables and fruits in the third position, and sugar in all its forms at the top tip is an additional advantage.

13. THE 7-DAY LOW-CARB RESCUE AND RECOVERY PLAN

The authors of this book are Drs. The book by Rachel and Richard Heller is hailed as the go-to resource for any low-carb dieter who wants assistance immediately getting back on track with any diet plan.

This book is for anybody who has had a crisis because of the holidays, a trip, a poor meal decision, or because they have hit an unfavorable weight loss plateau.

The physicians provide a 7-day food plan to help you get back on track and advise on stopping seeking carbohydrates, handling saboteurs, and spotting hidden sugars and carbs.

The Hellers begin by pointing out that persons who

are overweight and those who have a sweet tooth vary physically from naturally slim people and should quit blaming themselves for their weight issues. Understanding what your body needs to lose weight and what it should avoid doing can only speed up the process.

They recommend a 7-day diet that balances insulin levels, controls cravings, and puts the body back in fat-burning mode. Once this is finished, you may return to your preferred low-carb strategy with fresh knowledge on how to avoid frequent errors. Seven stages should be added every day. As follows:

- Every meal and snack should have a low-carb protein.
- Include salad and/or low-carb vegetables in your lunch, supper, and snacks.
- In proportion to any high-carb meals you may be eating, include a sizeable piece of low-carb protein, vegetables, and/or salad.
- Before consuming your high-carb item, finish all of your low-carb protein, vegetables, and salad.
- Eat only low-carb snacks. Keep high-carbohydrate items for meals.
- Eat solely low-carb items for one dinner and all snacks.
- Eat only low-carb items for your two meals and

all snacks.
You will be free to return to the low-carb diet of your choice if you have completed these steps over seven days. To assist you in sticking to your diet plan, they advise against using sugar alternatives like those included in diet sodas.

They also advise everyone who follows a low-carb diet to balance their meals' carbohydrate intake. In this manner, they begin to fill up on protein and reduce starch carbohydrates. Finally, you may consume the foods on your plate that are heavier in carbs and starch. You will feel fuller and eat less of the items that could be harming you as a result. Additionally, your body will be working so hard to break down the protein and fiber you ate that it won't have time to properly digest the high-carb meal once it has entered your system.

14. LOW-CARB LIFESTYLE

This book, whose rather lengthy subtitle promises to teach "everything food-loving dieters need to know to achieve lasting success, including: strategies for controlling binges and cravings, dealing with sudden weight gains, and secret metabolic weapons," was written by Fran McCullough, the author of The Low-Carb Cookbook.

This book is a supplement to the low-carb diet of your choosing and is meant to provide you with advice and strategies to make the transition to a low-carb lifestyle easier and less challenging.

This book explains how to make veggies taste like spaghetti and provides sources for low-carb bread and other treats. Additionally, there are hints for different cooking tools that might simplify your life and advice for filling a low-carb pantry.

McCullough also advises maintaining a low-carb diet while leading an active lifestyle. Examples include advice for traveling around Europe while hiking or camping. There are also recommendations on how to satisfy your carbohydrate cravings with low-carb alternatives.

For instance, she provides a straightforward recipe for potato skins and a pizza without a crust. Even a concept for an ice cream alternative that combines dairy and fruit exists.

While McCullough briefly reviews numerous low-carb diet fundamentals at the beginning of this book, she focuses more on providing recipes, suggestions, and methods. Don't seek diet fundamentals here.

CHAPTER 3

SUCCESS ADVICE

Dieting is difficult. If it were, we would all likely be in good shape. Successful individuals employ some weight loss strategies to help others because we are not.

SUCCESS TIP NO 1: DRINK 8–10 GLASSES OF WATER DAILY.

Okay, this is a significant issue for a lot of individuals. Generally speaking, water doesn't taste all that wonderful since it doesn't really "taste" like anything. The more often you do it, the simpler it is to drink eight to ten times daily. Simply training your taste senses and yourself to make it easy to accomplish is all required. Once you start, you'll start to want water.

The first thing you should do is drink a glass of water in the morning before breakfast. Remembering to drink water throughout the day will be easier since this is likely the simplest glass you will ever drink. Why not have two glasses instead?

Use a water-purifying pitcher or filter if you can't stand the taste of water. Add a few drops of lemon or lime to your water instead of sugar or other sweeteners. Ice is also useful.
Examine the flavored waters available on the market. Simply watch out for additives.

SUCCESS TIP NO. 2: EAT BREAKFAST

Avoid skipping breakfast. You should get up 20 minutes earlier every morning, so if you need to go to bed a bit earlier, do it! Breakfast is crucial for maintaining excellent health and a healthy weight. Your metabolism slows while you sleep, and it doesn't rev back up until you eat again, claims Dr. Barbara Rolls, a professor of nutrition at Penn State University.

Eating breakfast will help you lose weight overall and make it easier to stick to your diet for the rest of the day. Your likelihood of bingeing if you miss breakfast, have something sweet and in the "bread" category.

A few hard-boiled eggs and some high-fiber, low-starch fruit are always good to have on hand. Breakfast is the ideal time to eat fruit if you intend to do so at any point throughout the day.

SUCCESS TIP NO. 3: EAT AT LEAST 3 MEALS AND 2 SNACKS EVERY DAY

One of the most difficult changes to make maybe this one. You are, after all, busy! Your "full-plate" is already filled. When will you have enough time to think about eating more frequently?

Eating more often will boost your metabolism in the same way as eating breakfast would. Ensuring that your snacks are scheduled and taken regularly throughout the day may also reduce the amount of unhealthy carbohydrates you consume.

Making some healthy food selections and preparing a few healthy snacks and meals only requires a little planning time each morning before you go for the day at the grocery store and home. Simply refer to the convenient list of snacks and appetizers presented later for ideas.

SUCCESS TIP NO. 4: AVOID WHITE FOODS

This is one simple technique to keep in mind foods to avoid. Say no if it contains sugar, flour, potatoes, rice, or corn. It will be simpler to identify those rice cakes as an unhealthy, high-carb snack if you keep in mind this general guideline.

Always seek colored fruits and vegetables to replace the white ones with. Purchase leafy greens like kale and spinach, broccoli, lettuce, bell peppers, green beans, peas, apples, melons, oranges, and grapes.

In addition to being colorful, these meals are also rich in fiber, minerals, and significant antioxidants. Consuming colored fruits and vegetables will bring diversity to your diet and boost your health in other ways.

SUCCESS TIP NO. 3: EAT YOUR VEGGIES

It is quite simple to blame poor nutrition on a low-carb diet. Avoid giving in to this urge. It's a good idea to start trying various veggies if you've solely eaten potatoes for vegetables for the last five years. This is crucial for your general well-being and to prevent certain unpleasant consequences of eating insufficient fiber.

You may locate veggies you like eating if you work hard enough. Try grilling vegetables and using real butter while cooking to increase the taste. Additionally, you may look for new recipes online or in cookbooks.

Remember that two cups of simple salad greens only

contain roughly 5 grams of carbohydrates if you consume 40 grams or fewer carbohydrates each day.No excuse exists for you not to eat your vegetables.

SUCCESS TIP 6: MAKE AS MUCH OF YOUR FOOD AS POSSIBLE

Even while there are more and more restaurants with low-carb menu options, many of them still aren't the best options. Numerous recipes exist for rapid.

And simple dishes you may make at home yourself. Do this as often as you can.

You can better control hidden sugar and other processed foods if you prepare your meals, as you will know all the ingredients.

The long-term cost reduction is another advantage. Compared to dining at restaurants and fast food outlets, you will save substantially on every meal, even if you visit the grocery store more often.
Having your preferred fresh food options on hand can make it simpler to stay on a diet.

SUCCESS TIP NO. 7: BUY A GOOD SET OF FOOD STORAGE CONTAINERS

Planning your meals and snacks will be much simpler if you have food storage containers of different sizes available. Nuts, fruits, and vegetables may be easily prepared, separated, and stored for later use when purchased in bulk.

For instance, you could pre-slice your apples and eat them as snacks over a few days. Simply chop them, wash them in lemon or pineapple juice, and store them. This will be a simple snack that you can cook right away.

Prepare a lunch and bring it to work. Better still, prepare two snacks and your lunch for the office.

SUCCESS TIP NO. 8: EAT SOME PROTEIN AT EACH MEAL AND AS A SNACK

In addition to what has already been said, protein increases calorie expenditure. According to Jeff Hample, Ph.D., R.D., a representative for the American Dietetic Association, "Protein is made up mainly of amino acids, which are harder for your body to breakdown, so you burn more calories getting rid of them."

Just consider how consuming a protein-rich snack, such as a couple of slices of turkey, ham, or some string cheese, might assist in weight loss.
You will feel more satisfied after eating protein, which will reduce your desire for unhealthy snacks.

SUCCESS TIP NO 9: AFTER EVERY SNACK, DRINK A GLASS OF WATER

Ever feel hungry after having a handful or a normal serving of nuts? Try drinking water afterward. The water will make you feel full and avoid overindulgence. This will help you get 8 to 10 glasses of water daily.

After a snack, drinking water will also assist in removing the aftertaste from your tongue.
It may aid in reducing your want for more.

SUCCESS TIP NO 10: SLOW DOWN AND SAVOR YOUR MEALS

Don't get into the habit of eating while standing up or eating rapidly. Sit down and chew. You will feel full and more content if you take the time to taste your meal and chew it slowly.

Eating more slowly will make it easier for you to take

in the flavors of your meal, focus on what you are eating, and determine when you are satisfied.

SUCCESS TIP NO. 11: EAT YOUR LARGER MEALS FIRST AND SMALLER MEALS AFTERWARD, EATING

A substantial breakfast and a smaller supper will make you feel better and lose weight more quickly. You may also want to consume most carbohydrates earlier in the day, keeping a salad and lean animal protein for the evening.

You will feel fuller for longer and have fewer cravings for unhealthy snacks if you eat bigger meals when you are most active throughout the day.

SUCCESS TIP NO. 12: CONSIDER EATING SALMON OR MACKEREL FOR BREAKFAST

Yes, this may sound strange, but it's one method to get the beneficial Omega-3 fatty acids into your diet and add some variation to your everyday meals. After a few months, you could become bored with your usual breakfast of eggs and bacon, but switching to fish will offer you the protein and fish oils you need.

You could just have the cold leftover salmon the

following morning with dill sauce or use canned salmon or mackerel in croquettes as a better sausage option.

SUCCESS TIP NO. 13: USE LETTUCE LEAVES INSTEAD OF BREAD

Try eating lettuce leaves with your sandwiches and hamburgers instead of bread or buns; while it may seem strange at first, you'll undoubtedly come to enjoy it.

You may construct a great wrap sandwich using lettuce instead of the tortilla and bread, or you can build a double cheeseburger with onions, pickles, and tomato wrapped in a full lettuce leaf.
This will provide diversity to your diet while increasing your fiber consumption and healthy carbohydrates.

SUCCESS TIP NO 14: HAVE A FRUIT DESSERT

We can all agree that we sometimes need a sweet treat, but how can you satisfy your sweet tooth while maintaining a low-carb diet?

You could also try cottage cheese with sweet

pineapples or strawberries, which would be much better.

If your low-carb diet would let it, this is a sweet and delicious substitute for more sugary treats since berries are sweet and rich in fiber and minerals, and dairy products are high in protein.
The protein in the dairy products and the fiber in the fresh fruit will make these sweets more full, which is an extra advantage.

SUCCESS TIP NO 15: PURCHASE FRESH FRUIT INSTEAD OF SQUEEZED FRUIT

If you study the labels on the commercial juices available at your local grocery store, you will quickly learn that many contain very little genuine fruit juice. Fruit juice may be quite alluring as a substitute for soda, but just how healthy is it?

Why not skip the juice completely and eat a fresh piece of fruit? Fresh fruit not only has less sugar than juice but also provides fiber that benefits you and can help you feel filled longer. What you will discover is loads of sugar water and other additives.

SUCCESS TIP NO 16: GO EASY ON MEAL

SUBSTITUTIONS

Nearly every day, new meal replacement drinks and bars enter the market with claims to be healthy. Yet, virtually all of them contain hydrogenated oil and sugars, including Zone Perfect bars.

However, generally speaking, you don't want to indulge in a meal replacement smoothie or bar daily. The bars, in particular, may only be marginally healthier than a Snickers candy bar.

SUCCESS TIP NO 17: IF SOMETHING SEEMS TOO GOOD TO BE TRUE, IT PROBABLY IS

You can buy premade low-carb foods with the label "low carb" in your local grocery store and numerous specialized stores that cater to the low-carb lifestyle, but that doesn't mean you should.

Although low-carb pastries may be alluring, remember that they still include wheat and sugar or a sugar substitute, which are common carbohydrate sources.

As an occasional treat, they could be healthier than your regular muffin, but keep in mind to adhere to the fundamentals for continuing success with low-carb eating.

SUCCESS TIP NO 18: CHOOSE ITEMS IN THE OUTSIDE AISLES AT THE GROCERY STORE

If you recognize the one feature that unites all grocery store layouts: the healthier goods are on the perimeter aisles, maintaining your low-carb diet will be simpler. Consider how the nutritious items—fruits, vegetables, meats, and dairy products—are organized along the walls of the grocery store.

The majority of the things you need for a low-carb diet can be found on the perimeter of the grocery store, except the few shops that offer butter and cheese in the middle near the frozen foods.
It will be much simpler to avoid carb cravings and fill your basket with nutritious foods if you learn to start on one end of the outer aisle and work your way around.

SUCCESS TIP NO 19: SPEND MONEY ON QUALITY COOKBOOKS

You will be astonished at the amount of low-carb and low-carb-friendly dishes you can discover in your normal Betty Crocker Cookbook. Granted, not all recipes in a cookbook are low-carb cuisine, but you need some variety in your diet.

Cookbooks are excellent resources that often provide helpful advice on selecting meat cuts and cooking meats, fruits, and vegetables in novel and fascinating ways.

Use these resources to try something new, interesting, and tasty, and remember that new low-carb recipes often appear on the market.

SUCCESS TIP NO 20: TAKE A QUALITY MULTIVITAMIN

Even the most careful food combiner may overlook certain beneficial vitamins, minerals, and trace elements in their meals since we can't all do it properly all the time. To ensure you receive all you need, consider taking a decent multivitamin.

However, the longer you eat low-carb and the more red meat you consume, the less anemia will be an issue, and you should be able to take vitamins with less iron. Check with your doctor first for suggestions, and you should be checked for anemia to determine whether you need a vitamin with iron.

Remember to stick to the low-carb diet plan that is perfect for you and add some variety to your meals to help you remain true to your health and weight reduction objectives. Your success is entirely up to you, assuming you are otherwise healthy.

CHAPTER 4

RECIPES AND FOOD IDEAS FOR TRAVELERS

Finding tasty and affordable snack options is one of the difficulties with low-carb diets, especially if you are on a tight budget and cannot afford special prepackaged foods. Another challenge with low-carb snacking and meal preparation is finding tasty ingredients that won't make you bored after a few days.

It is easy to focus on what foods are not allowed, and too often, that seems to be our main focus, but there are many quick meal and snack possibilities right in front of us if we just think about them creatively. Low-carb dieters need to be creative in their food choices.

Here are some ideas for quick meals and snacks on the go. Some foods, like chicken, can be eaten as a snack or as the basis for a filling meal. For example, chicken breast can be grilled and eaten with various low-starch, high-fiber vegetables for a nutritious dinner. Sliced cold chicken breast can also make an enticing snack on the go.

Enjoy these meals alone as snacks or as part of a main dish, but make sure your choices are consistent with the low-carb diet of your choosing and that they are permitted at your stage in the plan:

APPETIZER AND SNACKS

String Cheese
Grapes
Apples
Dried Fruit
Canned Chicken
Canned Tuna
Proscuitto
Shrimp With Cocktail Sauce
Oranges
Peanut Butter
Edamame (Soybeans)
Celery Sticks
Humus
Garbanzo Beans (Chickpeas)
Hard Boiled Eggs
Low-Fat Yogurt
Low-Fat Milk
Unsweetened Apple Sauce
Sliced Turkey
Cherry Tomatoes
Baby Carrots
Cucumber With A Sugar-Free Dressing

Frozen Bell Pepper Slices
Beef Cold Roast
Bacon Strips
Jerky
Oysters
Sardines
Pork Rinds

BEVERAGES

FUNNY FRUITY

1 1/2 cups strawberry juice or strawberries
1/2 Cup Orange juice
1/4 cup Grapefruit juice
1 teaspoon of lemon juice
11/2 cups bottled (or tap) water
1 lb frozen white grapes with no seeds

Use frozen grapes as ice cubes and combine all ingredients in a big pitcher, except the grapes, before pouring and serving.

DELICIOUS TOMATO TREAT

2 cups of vegetable or tomato juice
2 tablespoons of lime juice
1 teaspoon Worcestershire sauce

1/2 tsp. horseradish
Several drops of our preferred hot sauce
Water-filled ice cube trays with lemon juice droplets are put onto each cube hole.

Combine all other ingredients in a pitcher, stir, and pour over lemon ice cubes. Place the ice cube tray in the freezer to set and create lemon-flavored ice cubes.

DESSERTS

WHIPPED JELLO TREAT

1 container of sugar-free Jello in your preferred flavor
2/3 cup of boiling water
2 cup ice cubes
1 container of thawed frozen whipped topping
Favorite nuts to taste

Boiling water is used to dissolve Jello. After pouring the mixture into a mixing bowl, add ice cubes and stir until the mixture thickens.

Stir quickly to incorporate the whipped cream, then pour into serving bowls and sprinkle with your choice of nuts.

DELISH PECANS

1/2 lb pecans
1 teaspoon cinnamon
1/2 sticks of melted margarine
Brown sugar, 1/4 cup

Pecans should be roasted for 10 minutes at 350 degrees.

Put the roasted nuts on a baking sheet, sprinkle with the cinnamon, brown sugar, and margarine, and bake for 10 minutes on each side, flipping once.

<u>MEAL TIME</u>

EASY ASPARAGUS OMELET WITH MUSHROOMS

2 eggs
2 tsp of water
3 steamed fresh asparagus spears
1/4 cup of white, sliced mushrooms
1/4 cup of reduced-fat mozzarella cheese, shredded

Pour the egg and water mixture into a small skillet lightly sprayed with nonstick cooking spray and heat over medium heat.

Once the top is hard, the top half of the omelet with asparagus, mushrooms, and cheese before covering it with the other half and serving.

CHEESY GARLIC AND CHEESE BROCCOLI

1 pound Broccoli florets
2 cloves minced garlic
2 tablespoons extra virgin olive oil,
1/4 cup freshly shredded cheese of your choice

After 2 minutes of steaming broccoli in 2 inches of water, drain it. Heat olive oil in a skillet over medium heat, stirring it to cover the bottom of the pan. Add the garlic, and cook it for approximately 1 minute or until it is fragrant.

After approximately 4 minutes of frequent tossing, add the broccoli and remove the pan from the heat. Add the cheese and gently mix.

GREEN BEANS AND BUTTERED ALMONDS

3 Tbsp. butter
1 pound of green beans
, salt and pepper to taste

Green beans should be boiled in a small amount of salted water for approximately 5 minutes, drained, and then sauteed with nuts and butter in a pan for 2 minutes while turning continuously.

CAULIFLOWER IN CREAM

1 pound Cauliflower florets
1/4 cup grated cheese, preferably Parmesan.
1 Tbsp soft butter
1/4 cup whipped cream
1/4 tsp. Salt
1/8 tsp. pepper

Cauliflower should be steamed in 2 inches of water for approximately 18 minutes or until soft, adding more water as needed.

Puree the cauliflower in a food processor or blender; add the other ingredients; mix until combined; transfer to a covered dish; chill; reheat over low heat.

MEATBALLS

1 pound of chicken
1/2 a pound of ground pork
1 egg

1 small onion, finely chopped
2 cloves minced garlic
2 tablespoons of dill
2 tbsp. Canola oil
Pepper and salt as desired

Combine all ingredients EXCEPT the oil in a bowl, and bake at 375 degrees.

Make roughly 12 meatballs from the ingredients by mixing everything well.

Meatballs should be browned in oil over medium heat before being transferred to a baking sheet or cookie jar and baked for 15 minutes or until well done.

SLOPPY JOES

1 pound ground beef
2 Tablespoons of finely sliced onion
salt and pepper to taste
1/2 tsp. of garlic
1 cup of smashed tomatoes
3 tablespoons brown sugar
1 teaspoon Worcestershire sauce
lettuce leaves or low-carb buns (or at least something other than white!)

Serve on (whole wheat or multi-grain) buns or lettuce leaves after the beef has been browned, drained, and cooked for approximately 10 minutes over low heat with the other ingredients.

STUFFED CHICKEN

4 skinless, boneless chicken breasts that have been cut in half
Parmesan cheese to taste
1 cup of chicken broth
1/2 cup of chopped mushrooms
2 teaspoons of chopped roasting red sweet pepper
1 tablespoon of water
1 clove minced garlic
1 teaspoon frying oil
1/4 teaspoon crushed dried marjoram

When mushrooms are soft and delicate, prepare to stuff them with garlic, pepper, and marjoram in a pan coated with nonfat cooking spray.

Create a pocket in the chicken pieces by cutting a slit through them. Fill the pocket with the freshly produced stuffing, then top with cheese (and, if you'd like, attach with toothpicks).

Chicken should be browned on all sides in a pan while

frying in oil. Add stock and simmer over medium to low heat until the chicken is no longer pink.

RESOURCES

Find out more about the low-carb lifestyle and featured diets in the following books:

Books:

350 Low Carb Cookbook: Quick and Delicious Low Carb Recipes Can Help You Lose Weight Effortlessly

DIETING AND WEIGHT LOSS: 5 Unexpected Dieting and Weight Loss Tips

Coconut Oil: Discover The Amazing Benefits of Coconut Oil From Skin Care, Hair Moisturizing, Weight Loss, Digestive Aid, Immune System Booster, & More........

CBD HEMP OIL: Use Hemp Oil To Look Better and Feel Better

Pure Yoga: Mastering The Healing Art For Health And Peacefulness

TOP KETOGENIC DIET: The Quickest & Easiest Way To weight loss

14 Days: To A Better KETOGENIC, DIET

A Guide To KETO, DIETING At Any Age: A Perfect Guide to Losing Weight, Boost Your Energy and Eating Healthy

The Untapped Gold Mine Of DIET, WEIGHT LOSS : That Virtually No One Knows About

Delicious And Healthy Diabetic Recipes: Over 500 Tasty And Healthy Recipes To Take Care Of Your Well-Being Without Sacrificing

Super Health For Super Kids: Parenting Guides For Picky Eating And Stronger Immune System
Respect All Life: Tasty Vegetarian Food And Cooking
Healthy Juicing: Exploring the Science, Nutrition, and Impact of Juicing on Your Health and Well-being

About The Author

Jennifer Schwarz is the owner and creator of kenvi Consulting, which offers various services to help you be as successful as possible. She's passionate about helping people get healthy and happy. Jennifer loves yoga, music, and teaching people how to be their best selves. She's also the writer behind Pure Yoga: Mastering the healing art for Health and Peacefulness, Organize your life: A most efficient method to organize your life, The untapped gold mine of diet, weight loss, and many more.

She is not a nutritionist or trained chef, just a determined mom who searched high and low for a way of eating that would reduce inflammation and allow her to live a happy and healthy life.

Jennifer lives in Dallas, Texas, with her husband and two beautiful children.

One Last Thing...

Dear Reader,

I hope you enjoyed reading this book and found it to be valuable for your needs. As an author, it means a lot to me when readers take the time to leave a review on Amazon. Your feedback not only helps me improve my writing but also helps potential readers decide if this book is right for them.

If you have a few minutes to spare, I would greatly appreciate it if you could leave a review on Amazon. Your honest opinion can help other readers make informed decisions and can make a real difference in the success of this book.

To leave a review, simply search for the book title and my name on Amazon.com, and select the book from the search results. Once you have navigated to the book's page, scroll down to the review section and share your thoughts on the book.

Rest assured that every single review is personally read and appreciated by me. Your feedback is crucial in helping me understand what worked well and what could be improved upon in future editions. Thank you in advance for your support and for taking the time to leave a review.

Best regards,

Jennifer Schwarz